Castor

A Beginner's Quick Start Guide on Hair Growth and Hair Loss Prevention Recipes

Copyright © 2022 Felicity Paulman

All rights reserved

No part of this book may be reproduced, or stored in a retrieval system, or transmitted in any form or by any means, electronic, mechanical, photocopying, recording, or otherwise, without express written permission of the publisher.

Printed in the United States of America

Disclaimer

By reading this disclaimer, you are accepting the terms of the disclaimer in full. If you disagree with this disclaimer, please do not read the guide.

All of the content within this guide is provided for informational and educational purposes only, and should not be accepted as independent medical or other professional advice. The author is not a doctor, physician, nurse, mental health provider, or registered nutritionist/dietician. Therefore, using and reading this guide does not establish any form of a physician-patient relationship.

Always consult with a physician or another qualified health provider with any issues or questions you might have regarding any sort of medical condition. Do not ever disregard any qualified professional medical advice or delay seeking that advice because of anything you have read in this guide. The information in this guide is not intended to be any sort of medical advice and should not be used in lieu of any medical advice by a licensed and qualified medical professional.

The information in this guide has been compiled from a variety of known sources. However, the author cannot attest to or guarantee the accuracy of each source and thus should not be held liable for any errors or omissions.

You acknowledge that the publisher of this guide will not be held liable for any loss or damage of any kind incurred as a result of this guide or the reliance on any information provided within this guide. You acknowledge and agree that you assume all risk and responsibility for any action you undertake in response to the information in this guide.

Using this guide does not guarantee any particular result (e.g., weight loss or a cure). By reading this guide, you acknowledge that there are no guarantees to any specific outcome or results you can expect.

All product names, diet plans, or names used in this guide are for identification purposes only and are the property of their respective owners. The use of these names does not imply endorsement. All other trademarks cited herein are the property of their respective owners.

Where applicable, this guide is not intended to be a substitute for the original work of this diet plan and is, at most, a supplement to the original work for this diet plan and never a direct substitute. This guide is a personal expression of the facts of that diet plan.

Where applicable, persons shown in the cover images are stock photography models and the publisher has obtained the rights to use the images through license agreements with third-party stock image companies.

Table of Contents

Disclaimer	3
Introduction	6
What Is Castor Oil?	7
Benefits of Castor Oil	9
Side Effects of Castor Oil	15
Ways to Use Castor Oil	18
Sample DIY Castor Oil Recipes	22
DIY Castor Oil	23
Homemade Castor Oil Pack	25
Scalp Nourishment Treatment Oil	28
Hair Growth Serum	29
Natural Hot Oil Hair Treatment	31
Castor Oil and Sugar Body Scrub	33
Castor Oil Massage	34
Organic Oil Cleanser	35
Castor Oil Facial Sleep Serum	37
Natural Lip Roller Blend	38
Conclusion	39
FAQ about Castor Oil	40
References and Helpful Links	42

Introduction

Castor oil is a type of vegetable oil that is made by pressing the seeds of the castor bean plant to extract the oil. The plant is indigenous to both Africa and India and has a long history of use as a traditional treatment for a wide range of illnesses across both continents.

It has seen a surge in popularity in recent years as a natural therapy option for a variety of diseases, including joint pain and constipation. Castor oil is known for its ability to reduce inflammation and also contains a high concentration of minerals and antioxidants. In addition to that, it can be found in a wide range of cosmetic items like soaps and lotions.

In addition, the use of castor oil has been shown to promote the overall health of hair. It is a natural conditioner that can contribute to giving the appearance of lustrous and shining hair. In addition, using castor oil on your hair can help prevent it from the damage that can be caused by environmental and heat styling causes.

In this quick beginner's guide, we will take a look at:

- What castor oil is
- What are its benefits
- What are its side effects
- How to use castor oil
- How to use it for hair growth and health

What Is Castor Oil?

Castor oil is made by pressing the seeds of the castor bean plant to extract the oil (Ricinus communis). Castor oil is a liquid that is colorless but has a hint of yellow to it, and it has been utilized in a wide number of applications for many years. It can be found functioning as a component in a wide variety of home goods, including paints and cleaning products.

Castor oil has been utilized historically in the treatment of a variety of medical disorders, most notably digestive problems. Castor oil is a natural laxative that you can use to help ease the discomfort of constipation. In addition to this, it is believed to strengthen the immune system, reduce inflammation, and enhance circulation.

It has a long history of use as a medicinal treatment, and more recently, it has gained favor as a natural beauty treatment. The oil has a high concentration of monounsaturated fatty acid known as ricinoleic acid. These kinds of fats have a reputation for being very good moisturizers. When they are applied to the skin, they help to prevent dryness and lock in moisture at the same time.

In addition, castor oil is a naturally occurring chemical that can assist in maintaining a healthy balance of oil production on the scalp and stimulate the development of hair. The hair follicles receive a significant amount of nourishment from the oil, which in turn promotes healthy development. Additionally, it might assist in giving the appearance of lustrous and shiny hair. In addition to this, it can shield the hair from the damage that is brought on by environmental and heat-styling elements.

Where to buy castor oil

Castor oil can be purchased in physical locations as well as on the internet. You may find it in the section of the store devoted to beauty products in almost any drug store or supermarket. Castor oil is also available to buy online from several different shops.

When shopping for castor oil, you should always opt for a product that has been extracted using a cold pressing method and is completely unadulterated. You may rest assured that you will receive an item of superior quality if you do this. Additionally, you should stay away from any items that have been processed or mixed with other oils.

Benefits of Castor Oil

Castor oil is a valuable treatment that can be put to a wide variety of applications because of its versatility and efficiency. It can confer significant health benefits when used appropriately. Castor oil is an all-natural solution that can be used for several different purposes, so it could be a nice option for you to consider.

Natural Laxative: Castor oil has a long history of use as a natural laxative that dates back many centuries. Castor oil is effective because it stimulates the muscles in the intestines, which in turn helps move waste through the digestive tract. In addition to this, it helps to soften stools and lubricates the intestines, which is very beneficial.

Here's how it works:

Castor oil contains ricinoleic acid, which is transformed into prostaglandin E2 by the body (PGE2). PGE2 is a molecule that helps induce contractions in the gut muscles and is known by its chemical name prostaglandin E2. The movement of trash through the digestive tract is assisted by these contractions.

When it is consumed first thing in the morning on an empty stomach, castor oil is at its most potent. The suggested serving size is one to two tablespoons. When consuming castor oil, it is essential to consume a lot of water because it has the potential to make one feel dehydrated. Although castor oil is usually seen to be safe for consumption, it has been linked to several adverse effects, including abdominal cramping, diarrhea, and nausea.

It can help to fight inflammation: Castor oil has been used to treat a wide array of conditions for many years. This is probably because of its unusual composition, which consists of ricinoleic acid, a type of fatty acid, among other components. It has been established that this fatty acid possesses anti-inflammatory qualities, which makes it an attractive option for the treatment of illnesses such as arthritis and joint pain. Castor oil helps to reduce inflammation and speed up the healing process when it is applied topically to the skin.

If you have sensitive skin, you should perform a patch test on a small area before using the oil all over. You can also dilute the oil by combining it with an equal amount of another carrier oil, such as jojoba or coconut oil. This is another method for reducing the potency of the oil.

Oral administration is another available option; however, before doing so, it is essential to consult a qualified medical practitioner. Before using castor oil, it is necessary to discuss the use of the product with your healthcare professional, particularly if you are pregnant or breastfeeding.

It can improve circulation: The most prevalent application for castor oil is in the treatment of circulatory issues in the legs, including varicose veins and peripheral artery disease. Other circulation-related illnesses, such as Raynaud's disease and frostbite, may also benefit from its use as a treatment option.

Castor oil can be used to improve circulation by simply massaging the afflicted area for ten to fifteen minutes with castor oil. You can perform this action once or twice each day, depending on your needs. You can also take a warm bath, add a few drops of castor oil to the water, and then soak in the water for twenty to thirty minutes.

Castor oil should only be used under the supervision of a medical professional if you have any preexisting medical conditions. Before applying it to a larger area of your skin, you should first make sure that you are not allergic to it by performing a patch test on a smaller area of your skin.

It can boost the immune system: Since ancient times, people have turned to castor oil as a natural treatment for a wide range of illnesses. Recently, it has been gaining popularity as a method to strengthen one's immune system, and this trend is expected to continue.

There is some evidence from scientific research that suggests castor oil could be beneficial for this objective. Castor oil was shown to have the ability, according to the findings of one study, to stimulate the formation of white blood cells. White blood cells are essential for the body's ability to fight off infections.

Castor oil is known to contain qualities that assist in reducing inflammation and fighting bacteria, both of which may contribute to further immune system enhancement.

If you are thinking about giving castor oil a shot in the hope that it may strengthen your immune system, you must discuss your plans with a qualified medical expert beforehand. They will be able to advise you on the most effective strategy to utilize while also ensuring that it is risk-free for you to do so.

Skincare: Since ancient times, people have turned to castor oil as a natural treatment for a wide range of illnesses. In more recent times, it has become increasingly popular as a natural approach to the maintenance of healthy skin.

The following is a list of benefits that castor oil may provide to the skin:

- It can help to soothe and heal inflamed skin by reducing redness and swelling.
- It can help to keep your skin hydrated by sealing in moisture.
- It can help to protect your skin from environmental damage by creating a barrier against harmful toxins and pollutants.
- It can help to reduce the appearance of wrinkles and fine lines by boosting collagen production.
- It can help to treat acne by unclogging pores and reducing inflammation.

Castor oil can provide these benefits if it is massaged into the skin after being applied to the afflicted area.

Depending on your requirements, you can perform this action once or twice every day.

If you have sensitive skin, you might want to dilute the castor oil with another carrier oil such as jojoba oil or almond oil. This is especially important if you use castor oil on your hair.

You can also get cosmetic goods like soaps, lotions, and creams that are formulated with castor oil. However, make sure you give the product's label a thorough read before using it to ensure that it is appropriate for the type of skin you have.

Taking care of your skin with castor oil is a risk-free and highly efficient method. If you have any concerns, however, you should discuss the matter with your primary care physician before utilizing this or any other natural cure.

Haircare: Castor oil is a natural product that may be worth experimenting with if you are searching for a way to help take care of your hair and stimulate the growth of new hair. Castor hail is an effective treatment for dandruff, split ends, and breakage that also stimulates the growth of new hair and enhances the overall condition of your hair. In addition to this, it helps to strengthen the hair follicles and gives the appearance of thicker, fuller hair.

Castor oil can be massaged into the scalp, or it can be applied directly to the hair if you prefer. Either way, it will benefit your hair. In addition to this, you can incorporate it into your shampoo or conditioner, or combine it with other oils such as olive oil or coconut oil.

If you want to see the maximum benefits of using castor oil to stimulate hair growth, you will need to apply it consistently. After a few weeks of consistent use, you should start to observe the effects of the product.

Side Effects of Castor Oil

Castor oil is a multipurpose and powerful natural medication due to its wide range of applications and associated health benefits. To cure a wide range of problems, including hair loss, skin disorders, and constipation, it can be either orally or applied topically to the affected area. When used correctly, castor oil is safe for the vast majority of individuals; nevertheless, some people may experience negative effects. If you see any of these negative effects, you should immediately stop using castor oil and talk to a medical professional.

Diarrhea: Castor oil is a traditional medication for the treatment of constipation that is derived from the beans of the castor plant. Castor oil has been used for several years. On the other hand, it has a strong laxative effect and, if taken in excessive amounts, can lead to diarrhea.

Castor oil is effective because it helps to stimulate the digestive tract and encourage regular bowel motions. Castor oil may have an adverse reaction to some medications, and it may not be appropriate for everyone to take it. Therefore, it is essential to see a medical practitioner before beginning to take castor oil.

Nausea: Even while castor oil is generally considered to be harmless, there is a possibility that some individuals can experience nausea after consuming it. If the castor oil is taken on an empty stomach, there is a greater chance of experiencing this unwanted side effect. Castor oil should ideally be consumed with food or drink to reduce the likelihood of experiencing nausea. If you find that you are feeling sick to your stomach, consider having a glass of ginger ale or eating a light snack. These home remedies may assist in calming your stomach and relieving any discomfort that you may be experiencing.

Stomach cramps: Stomach pains are one of the negative side effects of using castor oil. The oil may cause the muscles in your bowel to tighten, which will result in cramping and pain. Diarrhea is a possible complication in some circumstances. You must get medical treatment if you develop any kind of abdominal pain after consuming castor oil.

Low blood pressure: Castor oil has several potential adverse effects, but one of the most noticeable is a drop in blood pressure. This is a result of the oil's ability to relax the blood vessels, which in turn helps to enhance blood flow. As a direct consequence of this, people who already have low blood pressure may have symptoms such as dizziness or lightheadedness when they use castor oil.

Pelvic Congestion: Castor oil can lead to pelvic congestion if it is consumed in excessive quantities. If you ingest an excessive amount of castor oil, you may get tightness in your pelvic region. It is possible to suffer from a condition known as pelvic congestion, which manifests itself when the veins in the pelvis become enlarged and uncomfortable. This can lead to several uncomfortable symptoms.

Allergic reactions: Castor oil is generally considered to be harmless; nevertheless, some individuals may have an adverse reaction to it. Itching, swelling, and difficulty breathing are some of the symptoms that might accompany an allergic reaction. If you suffer any of these symptoms, you should immediately stop using the oil and seek professional medical help.

Ways to Use Castor Oil

Castor oil is extracted from the beans of the castor plant and has a long history of usage as a traditional cure for a wide range of ailments across several different medical specialties. Constipation, skin problems, and joint discomfort are still some of the conditions that it is used to treat today.

Many different applications are possible for castor oil. It can be ingested orally, applied topically, or administered via an enema to achieve the desired effect.

Orally: Castor oil can induce regular bowel movements and help loosen stools when it is consumed in the form of food. It is essential to begin treatment with a low dose of castor oil and to gradually raise this dose as directed. You can also get castor oil in capsule form, and you can take these capsules with either food or liquid. Because they are simpler to consume than the oil itself, some people choose to take supplements in the form of capsules.

If you are pregnant or breastfeeding, you should not consume castor oil in any form. There has not been enough research done to determine whether or not it is safe. Castor oil should be used in decreasing doses at the beginning of treatment to reduce the risk of negative effects. To avoid being dehydrated, it is essential to consume a large amount of water whenever one takes castor oil by mouth. Castor oil should be discontinued immediately and medical attention sought if any adverse reactions occur while using it.

If you are considering using castor oil as a treatment for a health condition, it is in your best interest to first consult with your healthcare professional so that you can go over the potential downsides and upsides of this treatment.

Topically: Castor oil has anti-inflammatory, analgesic, and wound-healing properties, and it can be used topically to provide these benefits. Additionally, it can be utilized as a moisturizer or oil for massages. Castor oil can be applied directly to the skin by simply massaging a tiny bit into the afflicted area after using the oil. It is recommended that you wait at least half an hour before rinsing off the oil to achieve the optimum results. To boost the effectiveness of your go-to lotion or cream, you can also incorporate a few drops of castor oil into the formulation.

Enema: The process of administering liquids into the rectum and colon through the anus is referred to as an enema. Castor oil is a common ingredient in enemas because of its efficacy in promoting regular bowel movements. Castor oil has emollient and lubricating properties, making it an excellent choice for anyone concerned about their digestive health.

It is essential to use a regular syringe and to inject the castor oil into the colon in a calm and measured manner when using castor oil in an enema. To accomplish this task most effectively, lie on your left side with your left leg extended and your right knee bent. It is essential to wait at least half an hour after the oil has been kept in place before departing. After the enema, you should take some time to relax.

Using it for hair growth and health

Castor oil has a variety of positive effects on hair, including the promotion of new hair development, the prevention of damage to existing hair, the hydration of the hair, the enhancement of its shine and fullness, and the enhancement of its general health. It can minimize frizz and mend split ends when applied to the ends of your hair in the same step.

It is essential to select a high-quality product when looking to stimulate hair growth with castor oil. Castor oil should ideally be organic, cold-pressed, and one hundred percent pure. This particular variety of castor oil is the most powerful and will bring about the desired effects in the shortest amount of time. Castor oils that have been treated with chemicals or heated should be avoided since these might cause your hair to get damaged.

To use castor oil for hair growth:

1. Start by heating the oil so it's warm but not hot.

2. Apply it to your scalp and massage it for several minutes.

3. Wrap your head in a towel or shower cap and leave the oil in for at least 15 minutes.

4. Wash your hair as usual.

5. For best results, repeat the process 6-8 times per week.

Consider utilizing castor oil if you're seeking a method that's more in line with nature to stimulate hair growth.

This simple treatment has been around for centuries and is quite affordable. It has been shown to stimulate new hair growth and enhance overall hair health. When used consistently, it has the potential to assist you in achieving thicker, fuller, and healthier hair.

Sample DIY Castor Oil Recipes

There are different recipes you can try using castor oil, depending on what benefits of the oil you wish to take advantage of. For starters, you can purchase castor oil in-store or online. You can also try to make your own if you're able to source the ingredients. Below is a castor oil DIY recipe, followed by other recipes to maximize the benefits you can get from castor oil as well as other essential oils.

DIY Castor Oil

Ingredients:

- castor seeds
- water

Instructions:

1. Prep the seeds by removing the shell, either by using hands or a machine.

2. Leave it dry out in the sun for about 7 hours. If using an oven, set it to about 60°C for 7 hours.

3. Transfer seeds onto a preheated pan over heat.

4. Roast the seeds by stirring continuously for about 2-3 minutes or until they are slightly brownish.

5. Use a mortar and pestle to grind the seeds until it turns into a paste. If you have access to a cold press machine, go ahead and use it.

6. Transfer the castor paste into a pan and add water. Set the heat to high.

7. Leave it to boil for about 4-5 hours, or until the oil floats on the surface.

8. The oil can now be scooped up using a spoon. However, experts recommend leaving the pan to cool overnight after boiling it before scooping it up.

9. Store the oil in a bottle.

Homemade Castor Oil Pack

Ingredient:

- castor oil

Materials:

- cotton flannel or wool, unbleached, cut into 10x12-inch or smaller strips, depending on preferred size

- plastic sheets, either from a clean trash bag or a small tablecloth

- scissors

- tongs

Instructions:

1. In a medium-sized bowl or container, pour castor oil. Make sure that the cloth can soak completely in it.

2. Soak a piece of cloth and pick it up with tongs. Make sure it's dripping with castor oil.

3. Transfer the soaked cloth onto the plastic sheet.

4. Repeat the process until you have three to four pieces of cloth of equal sizes.

5. Make sure that you put the cloth on top of each other. This stack of soaked cloths is your castor oil pack.

Application:

1. Place a towel or a sheet on where you'll lie down to catch any oil drips.

2. Put the castor oil pack on the body part that needs treating.

3. Top the pack with a plastic sheet, so you can press it against your skin while also heating the pack.

4. If preferred, you can apply more heat by placing a heating pad or hot water bottle on the plastic sheet. Just make sure that you don't leave this unattended to avoid burns.

5. Allow your castor oil pack to sit on your skin for about 45 to 60 minutes.

6. Remove the oil pack. Using a towel that's warm and damp, wipe off the area to clean excess oil.

7. Don't throw away the pack. Store it in a container where you can soak them again. Cover tightly.

8. Put it in the refrigerator. This castor oil pack can be reused up to 30 times.

Note:

- It's recommended that you use castor oil that is hexane free.

- Don't use the microwave to heat the castor oil pack.

- Avoid using the oil pack if you're pregnant or breastfeeding. It's still unclear if castor oil has effects on a baby, so it's best to avoid it now.

- Don't apply the oil pack on skin that is irritated, cut, scratched, or has open wounds. Also, avoid using the oil pack on injured body parts.

Scalp Nourishment Treatment Oil

Ingredients:

- 1 tbsp. castor oil
- 1 tbsp. unrefined virgin coconut oil
- 1 drop lavender essential oil
- 1 drop tea tree oil

Instructions:

1. In a glass bowl, pour castor oil and VCO together.

2. Prepare a double broiler to warm up the mixture, only until the VCO warms up.

3. Add the rest of the oils to warm up before removing the bowl from heat.

Application:

1. Use the oil while warm. Massage it gently on your scalp.

2. Let it sit on your scalp for about 30 to 60 minutes. You can also leave it overnight.

3. Use your usual shampoo and conditioner to wash the oil out of your hair.

Note:

- This is a great oil treatment for those who have dry, flaky scalp and hair.

Hair Growth Serum

Ingredients:

- 1 tbsp. castor oil
- 1 tbsp. argan jojoba oil
- 6 drops rosemary essential oil

Instructions:

1. Prepare a 1-oz. dropper bottle for this serum.

2. Pour all the ingredients into the bottle.

3. Shake well to blend all the oils.

Application:

1. Put two drops onto your fingertips.

2. Smoothen oil over the middle strands to the ends of the hair. You can do this to either dry or wet hair. No need to rinse.

Notes:

- This serum may be used before or after washing the hair, depending on the preference.

- This blend may also be used as a massage oil every week.

- Aside from the benefits of castor oil, rosemary essential oil is also a popular natural oil that promotes hair growth and helps with itchy scalp and dandruff by massaging into the scalp.

Natural Hot Oil Hair Treatment

Ingredients:

- 30 ml castor oil, organic
- 20 ml argan oil, organic
- 20 ml extra virgin olive oil, organic
- 30 g virgin coconut oil, organic
- 1 ml or about 20 drops rosemary oil, organic

Instructions:

1. In a microwave-safe bowl or beaker, pour in the castor oil, argan oil, EVOO, and VCO.

2. Heat the mixture in the microwave until the VCO melts.

3. Remove the oils from the microwave and pour the rosemary oil. Mix.

4. Transfer the oil into a dark-colored bottle with a cover. Label properly.

Application:

1. Allow the mixture to cool if it's a fresh batch before using.

2. Apply oil onto damp hair, coating the entire length of your hair strands from root to tip.

3. Use an old towel or shirt to cover your hair. Leave it for 30-60 minutes.

4. Wash off the oil with your usual shampoo and conditioner. It's advisable to shampoo your hair twice to rinse out all the oil.

5. Air dry your hair if possible.

Note:

- Using this mixture on damp hair helps the oil to properly penetrate the hair and locks in the moisture as it dries.

Castor Oil and Sugar Body Scrub

Ingredients:

- 1/4 cup castor oil
- 1 cup plain white or brown granulated sugar
- a few drops of essential oils*

Instructions:

1. Put the sugar into a pint-sized container or mason jar.

2. Gently add the castor oil while mixing.

3. Add a few drops of your preferred essential oil.

4. Keep your jar tightly covered. When using, make sure to not let water into it.

Notes:

- You can adjust the amount of castor oil depending on how saturated or dry you want it to be. For dryer consistency, either use less oil or add more sugar.

- You can use your favorite essential oils in this mixture. For a more relaxing scent, use ylang-ylang or lavender. Otherwise, use lemon or orange for an uplifting scent.

- Use a scooper whenever you're going to get some scrub from the jar, or scoop out a few before you bathe, to ensure that water won't get into the jar so as not to dissolve the sugar.

Castor Oil Massage

Ingredients:

- 3 tbsp. castor oil
- 3-4 drops bergamot essential oil
- 3-4 drops chamomile essential oil
- 5-6 drops lavender essential oil

Instruction:

Mix all the oils in a bottle and shake well.

Application:

1. Pour a few drops of the oil on your hands.

2. Apply on the neck and shoulders while massaging. Do this before going to sleep.

Organic Oil Cleanser

Ingredients:

- 15 ml castor oil, organic
- 34 ml coconut fractionated oil, organic
- 0.5 g high-strength vitamin E
- 0.5 ml or 8 drops grapefruit essential oil, organic

Instructions:

1. Pour out all the ingredients in a bowl or container to mix them well.

2. If you have a glass bottle, transfer the oil in there and cover. Add a label as well.

Application:

1. Get a cotton wool pad and apply a few drops of the cleansing oil.

2. Wipe your face and neck with the pad. If you're wearing makeup, repeat this process until everything is removed.

3. You can also skip using a cotton pad and use your fingers to apply the oil by massaging it all over your face.

4. Use a clean muslin cloth soaked in warm water to wipe off the oil-soaked makeup.

Note:

- Using an organic floral water rinse can also help tone your skin and remove any residual oil. Rose or lavender water is great. Just dab a few drops of floral water on a cotton pad and sweep it across your face. Make sure that you moisturize after.

Castor Oil Facial Sleep Serum

Ingredients:

- 1 tbsp. castor oil
- 1 tbsp. argan oil
- 1 tsp. rosehip seed oil
- 2 drops geranium essential oil

Instructions:

1. In a small container, mix castor, argan, and rosehip seed oils. Shake well.

2. Add the geranium essential oil. Mix.

Application:

Use this facial serum after cleansing and toning before going to bed.

Note:

- This is advisable for nighttime use because of the heavy oils.

Natural Lip Roller Blend

Ingredients:

- 1 tsp. castor oil
- 1 tsp. jojoba oil
- 1 drop frankincense essential oil
- 1 drop lavender essential oil

Instructions:

1. In a glass bottle, pour everything together.

2. Shake to blend everything smoothly.

Application:

1. Roll onto the lips anytime you feel like doing so.

2. Use the lip blend, especially during bedtime, to nourish your lips overnight.

 Note:

- If you can source a small roller bottle, use that. If not, you may use any other small bottles you have at home.

Conclusion

Castor oil is a vegetable oil that has been used for centuries for medicinal purposes. It is obtained by pressing the seeds of the castor plant, Ricinus communis. Castor oil is a colorless to very pale yellow liquid with a peculiar taste and odor. It is one of the oldest known medicines and has been mentioned in ancient Egyptian texts.

Castor oil is used in the treatment of various conditions, including constipation, skin disorders, and hair loss. It is also used as a laxative and can be taken orally or applied topically. Castor oil is safe for most people when used as directed.

However, side effects may occur, such as diarrhea, stomach cramps, and nausea. If you experience any of these side effects, stop using castor oil and consult your doctor. Castor oil is a versatile and effective remedy that can be used for many different purposes.

When used correctly, it can offer significant health benefits. If you're looking for an all-natural remedy with a variety of uses, castor oil may be a good option for you.

FAQ about Castor Oil

Q: What is castor oil?

A: Castor oil is a vegetable oil that has been used for centuries for medicinal purposes. It is obtained by pressing the seeds of the castor plant, Ricinus communis.

Q: What are the benefits of castor oil?

A: Castor oil is used in the treatment of various conditions, including constipation, skin disorders, and hair loss. It is also used as a laxative and can be taken orally or applied topically.

Q: What are the side effects of castor oil?

A: Side effects of castor oil may include diarrhea, stomach cramps, and nausea. If you experience any of these side effects, stop using castor oil and consult your doctor.

Q: How do I use castor oil?

A: Castor oil can be taken orally or with an enema and can be applied topically. It is important to follow the directions on the product label.

Q: Is castor oil effective for hair growth?

A: There is some anecdotal evidence that castor oil may promote hair growth, but more research is needed to confirm this. When used regularly, castor oil can help improve the overall health of your hair. However, it is important to consult with a doctor before using this oil if you are pregnant or nursing. Additionally, avoid using castor oil if you have an allergy to it.

Q: *Where can I purchase castor oil?*

A: Castor oil is available for purchase online and in stores. It can be found in the beauty aisle of most drug stores or supermarkets. You can also purchase castor oil online from a variety of retailers.

Q: *Is castor oil safe?*

A: Castor oil is safe for most people when used as directed. However, side effects may occur. If you experience any of these side effects, stop using castor oil and consult your doctor.

References and Helpful Links

8 creative uses for castor oil around the house. (2021, March 24). https://www.bobvila.com/slideshow/8-creative-uses-for-castor-oil-around-the-house-579372.

12 great health benefits of castor oil. (n.d.). The Times of India. Retrieved August 12, 2022, from https://timesofindia.indiatimes.com/life-style/health-fitness/diet/health-benefits-of-castor-oil/articleshow/40063531.cms.

30 outstanding castor oil uses and benefits | one agora health. (n.d.). Retrieved August 12, 2022, from https://www.oneagorahealth.com/30-outstanding-castor-oil-uses-and-benefits.html.

Benefits of castor oil for skin with diy recipes—Carrier oil spotlig. (n.d.). Retrieved August 12, 2022, from https://www.lovingessentialoils.com/blogs/healthy-living/benefits-of-castor-oil-for-skin-diy-recipes.

Castor oil: Benefits, use, and side effects. (2018, June 28). https://www.medicalnewstoday.com/articles/319844.

Clinic, A. S., Laser &. Wellness. (2016, March 17). 5 natural treatments for visible spider veins. https://alluraclinic.com/blog/natural-treatments-for-visible-spider-veins/

Diy castor oil packs and how to use them. (2019, December 17). https://www.healthline.com/health/castor-oil-pack.

Effective natural remedy to treat the effects of Raynaud's Syndrome. (2018, February 2). https://healthnwellness.co.uk/effective-natural-remedy-to-treat-the-effects-of-raynauds-syndrome/.

How castor oil can help moisturize your scalp and hair. (n.d.). Retrieved August 12, 2022, from https://www.verywellhealth.com/using-castor-oil-for-hair-growth-4172190.

How to make castor oil at home. (n.d.). Retrieved August 12, 2022, from https://www.youtube.com/watch?v=ttsfw7V3mXE.

Ihenacho, C. (2017, July 21). How to make castor oil. https://www.legit.ng/1115915-how-castor-oil.html.

p-themes. (n.d.). Easy castor oil recipes. Retrieved August 12, 2022, from https://naissance.com/blogs/naissance-blog/easy-castor-oil-recipes.

University, C., & University, S. (n.d.). How to use castor oil for skin: Easy diy recipes. Retrieved August 12, 2022, from https://www.treehugger.com/castor-oil-for-skin-5199433.

User, S. (n.d.). Four amazing beauty benefits of castor oil. Retrieved August 12, 2022, from https://www.longevitymed.com/blog/four-amazing-beauty-benefits-of-castor-oil.html.

Milton Keynes UK
Ingram Content Group UK Ltd.
UKHW021308270823
427563UK00023B/794